QUIET

Use Your Quiet Life, Inner Strength and Power For Your Guide To Success

Published by WOS WorldWide Publishing

First Printing, 2013

ISBN-13:978-0615910000
ISBN-10:0615910009

Printed in the United States of America

Introduction

The world views powerful people to be those who are out-spoken, energetic and charismatic—the extroverts. Most often time, extroverts are seen as the smartest in the class and have the greatest potential. Would you believe that not all great people are extroverts? What would you say if I told you that some of the most influential women in history are not extroverts, but in fact *introverts*? Rosa Parks, Eleanor Roosevelt, and Mother Teresa are just a few phenomenal female introverts who have shaped the world into what we know it is today. While these women were quiet and reserved, they commanded attention when the need arose. They used their quietness and thoughtfulness to their advantage. And the world listened.

When people think of introverts, they usually use the terms; shy, aloof, quiet, and even arrogant! These terms can be offensive if said to the wrong introvert. People often times think that introvert and shy are synonymous and can be interchangeable. They aren't. Shy folk can be handicapped by their fear of social interactions—large or small—whereas people who are introverted simply do not need to be in the lime-light all the time. They can command attention when the need arises; however, just be sure to give them some breathing room after the need passes. Unlike extroverts who are instantly out looking for their next "high," an introvert simply needs to be able to decompress and collect their thoughts.

Some notable characteristics of introverts are that they are very thoughtful and observant. These people take in their surroundings and watch others. They are able to process what they see in ways that an extrovert may not be able to. An introvert has the ability to see the larger picture when it comes to situations, and because of their keen observations and processing, they can make well informed and well thought out decisions. These decisions can be very important and maybe even lucrative! Where extroverts make decisions based on impulse and emotion, an introvert will take into consideration all the facts presented and weigh the pros and cons of each choice. You could think of it this way, an introvert can rule the world because they can see what is good for the many, not just the few.

There are discussions in the scientific world regarding introverts and extroverts. Studies have been done comparing the quality of life two personality types. Some would suggest that an extrovert tend to lead a happier, more successful life, however that isn't always true. Introverts often times enjoy their solitude and find great contentment in their smaller group of friends. Like the women of history that was mentioned before, introverts can act extroverted for a while; they can even find enjoyment in this. But when all is said and done, the real enjoyment comes when the event is over and they are alone and are able to reflect. Reflection, solitude, quiet contemplation and deep thinking are words that can be summarize any introverted person.

Contents

Introvert or Just Shy?

What Is An Introvert?

You're at a party and you are approached by someone of the opposite sex. Suddenly your heart is racing and you develop a self-conscious clumsiness. Introverted or shy? Conversely, your friend is at the same party. She seems to be comfortable as she makes the rounds, visiting with friends and meeting new people. Then, suddenly she's at your side. The party seems to be just getting lively, but she's ready to leave. Again, introverted or shy?

Clearly there is a difference in the way the two individuals in this scenario react and interact with people. The first instance describes a shy person, someone who suffers from anxiety at being in large groups, meeting members of the opposite sex or generally being in a social situation. The second is a classic description of an introvert.

Many people think that introversion and shyness are one and the same. But they would be wrong. An introverted person does not normally fear a crowd or a social situation; they just value their alone time more than an extrovert would. In the above situation, the introverted person was not uncomfortable socializing at this party. She visited with friends and, for a period of time, seemed to enjoy herself. But there was a limit to her gregariousness. Suddenly, something changed; she had reached her "social saturation point," and wanted her peace and quiet back.

An introverted person does not dislike people; he or she simply has more of a craving for quiet time than the extravert. He needs time for introspection, to think and meditate. An introverted person is not normally drawn to situations in which they need to be "on" all the time. He is more in touch with his inner self. He is comfortable with the prospect of a quiet night at home, reading a good book or just enjoying the solitude.

Shyness is defined as a behavior. Being shy means being afraid in social situations. By comparison, introversion is described as a motivation. Introversion is determining how much time one wants or needs to spend in a social situation. Since introverts gather their energy and focus from within, it may be difficult for them to last very long in a social situation where they are called upon to interact with many different types of extroverted or changing personalities. They discharge their own personality energy at an enormous rate and may soon feel depleted and have a hard time focusing.

An extrovert, on the other hand, craves being with people. She needs external stimulation to be happy. There is nothing wrong with that. In fact, both introversion and extraversion are normal traits and require no apologies nor explanations. They are simply two opposite ends of a scale, with numerous variations in between. We are born with a leaning toward one or the other of these personality traits, just as we are born to some degree with a tendency toward shyness.

The difference between introversion and shyness is that shyness can be crippling and may interfere with our joy in living. Introversion does not. It is simply a preference. According to studies on the subject, we are all born with a degree of both introversion and extraversion, although naturally leaning more heavily toward one or the other.

There is an interesting website based on the Myers-Briggs Type Indicator (MBTI) that can help you determine where you fall in this scale between introvert and extravert. Based on just four questions, it characterizes your natural tendency in this regard. There are so many possible variations, it makes for a fascinating study. If you are curious as to where you fit into this personality scale, you can Google MBTI to analyze yourself.

Some of the common characteristics of an introvert are that they are thoughtful and self-aware, they are quiet and reserved in large groups (not to be confused with the shy person's reaction to the same); they are social beings, but require time alone to recharge; and they are generally observant people who seek self-knowledge. They also tend to be very private about expressing their emotions.

If introversion and shyness are so different, it makes one wonder why they seem to be so closely linked. Both the introverted person and the shy person tend to be quiet by nature, thus the introvert is often accused of being, or thought of as, shy. There are, however, introverts who lean heavily toward social situations, so they cannot all be lumped under the same label. Sadly, society tends to judge quiet people more harshly, no matter what the reason. Studies show we rank extroverts – the talkers, the social butterflies – as somehow more competent, more likable, and maybe even smarter. This is a grossly unfair assessment. It ignores the introvert's skills of analyzing a situation,, their self-awareness and craving for answers – clearly qualities indicating a great degree of intelligence.

The best example I can think of to demonstrate an introvert's thinking is a situation I myself was in recently. We had a young man stop by to pick up my son; they were going on a camping trip. When personalities were dished out, this young man seems to have gotten assigned a triple dose! He was charming and likable, charismatic and fun to be with – and clearly a Type A extrovert! I thoroughly enjoyed being with him – for about twenty minutes. Then, I could almost feel something click inside of me. I had had enough and just wanted them to be on their way. It was nothing personal, although I must say I would find it difficult to be so "on" all of the time!

I am undeniably a self—professed introvert.

Introverts are also often accused of being aloof and even arrogant. In an article in the Atlantic Monthly, writer Jonathan, Rauch theorizes that many of these misunderstandings result from the extravert's failure to understand how introverts function. While "extraverts have little or no grasp of introversion, they assume that ... their own [company] is always welcome. They cannot begin to fathom why anyone would prefer to be alone." As extraverts, they simply do not "get it"!

As a result of the combination of this craving to be alone and this mislabeling, it is not uncommon for introverts to have fewer friends, just a few choice people to which they feel particularly close. Compare this to the extrovert who has a wide circle of friends. Introverts prefer to interact with people one on one; or a small dinner party of maybe four to six guests rather than a large group. Within that small group of people, the introvert enjoys engaging inn challenging, meaningful conversations.

Introverts make up a much smaller portion of the population, but that does not mean they are a flawed group by any means. Introverts are the writers among us and computer programmers, artists and accountants. They are often the creative types.

Does Science Confirm That Extroverts Are Happier Than Introverts?

It is not true that extroverts are better than introverts, but studies have demonstrated that they generally feel happier. It seems as if our society needs both types of people. The quiet author is as revered as the outgoing politician, and maybe more so. But in fact, it is also true that introverts may get that same rush of happiness when they are called upon to act like extroverts. The quiet author might feel great after he does a book tour about his latest work. He may just take more time to reflect on the positives and negatives of the experience while he sits alone afterwards.

But in general, introverts and extroverts tend to process gratification differently. Even when introverts act like extroverts for a time, they tend to respond to the experience differently afterwards. While an extrovert might be looking for his next conquest, an introvert may take advantage of time alone to reflect upon his experiences. Their brains tend to process experiences differently.

Are Introverts More Realistic About The Past?

Introverts may need more time to process experiences because they are more realistic about the past. According to a psychological researcher at San Francisco State University, Ryan Howell, extroverts are happier because they tend to remember the past in a more positive light. In other words, they come equipped with a good pair of rose-colored glasses. He made this comment, based upon his studies, in a statement that was reported in Live Science here: http://www.livescience.com/13997-extrovert-nostalgia-fuels-happiness.html

He compared extroverts to neurotic people who tend to remember past events in the exact opposite way, by dwelling on the negatives of past events. That is not to say that introverts are neurotic though, but might simply have a more realistic view of events with both positive and negative aspects of the past being more clearly reflected upon. So it may be true that introverts are more honest with themselves, but certainly less positive than true extroverts. There are a lot of books about the power of positive thinking, and these may be intended to help introverts act more like extroverts so they can be happier people.

Are Introverts Happier When They Behave Like Extroverts?

This idea is supported by other studies. For example, there is the idea that introverts are actually happier when they are acting like extroverts, at least for a time. They get the same rush from having people respond to their opinions or work. They like attention and a feeling of being in control as well as anybody does. Well, actually they may not get the same rush. Extraverts might be more sensitive to feel-good chemicals in their brain. But introverts do get a rush too.

William Fleeson, a psychology professor at Wake Forest University, says that the same outgoing actions can make both introverts and extroverts happier than they might have been without those actions. He reported on his findings in The Journal of Personality in 2012.

This week-long study followed eighty-five subjects as they participated in different experiences and recorded their happiness levels on hand-held devices. At the end of this study, the responses and activities were collected, summarized, and reviewed.

Both introverts and extroverts recorded feeling happier when they were engaged in activities that are associated with extroverted behavior. These might be social events, presentations, or other group activities where the subject has some attention and control. Apparently, introverts reported feeling happier when they were behaving like extroverted people. These results have been supported by other studies too: You can read more about this here in the Wall Street Journal:
http://online.wsj.com/article/SB1000142412788732 4144304578621951399427408.html

Lots Of Introverts Say They Are Perfectly Happy

Some very successful introverts disagree with this study. They do say they feel a rush after giving a presentation, enjoying a comfortable social group, or participating in a similar activity. But they contend that they are quite happy when they are working on a book, reading, or taking a solitary walk. It might not be a rush of happiness, but it is contentment. They say the rush of elation is not what they really consider happiness, but may even be relief that the event is over and they can get back to what they truly love to do.

Do Introverts Simply Need More Time To Be Introspective?

Still, unhappy introverts might move out of their comfort zones more often. Because they tend to judge the past more harshly, they do not always have optimistic expectations about good ones. A psychology professor in the UK, Brian Little, says that introverts might also need more time recharge after extroverted activities, even if they enjoy them. For example, Dr. Little says he might enjoy giving a speech or participating in a conference. But while other group members might enjoy socializing after the activity, he would rather take a walk by himself to emotionally recharge and review the event.

There you go. It might just be that introverts need more time to recharge because part of the experience for them is the ability to be introspective about it. Extroverts would rather get positive feedback from other people. That said, nobody is a pure introvert or pure extrovert. Most people fall somewhere on the scale. It is also not easy to tell which category somebody falls into by the way they act in public. A better test might be the way a person acts after the public event is over.

Everybody has heard stories about famous actors or notable politicians who can command a crowd, but are really quite soft-spoken and shy when encountered in a one-on-one situation. This might be an example of introverts who are acting like extroverts because they need to for their profession.

This whole debate might force people to truly define happiness. Is it long-term contentment or a rush of elation. Introverts might view extroverts as unhappy because they always seem to be striving for their next opportunity to get a "fix" of attention or control. Introverts might regard this more like the icing on the cake, but not the true meal that keeps them content.

Why Being An Introvert Is A Good Thing:

When most people think of introverts, they think of them in a negative way. They imagine someone silent and brooding while living a life of solitude. While this may be the way of life for some people, there are others that have learned to use their introversion to their benefit. If you have no idea why this makes all of the sense in the world, you should probably continue reading.

Being understood when they speak is a great benefit that introverts have. They are not extremely verbose, so they tend to choose their words very carefully. The fact is that they would rather make sure that the listener gets the point the first time than having to repeat themselves. This cuts down on common miscommunication issues and makes it simpler for people to work with them.

It takes a lot of thought to rule the world, so introverts are definitely yards ahead of everyone else. While extroverts speak out of turn and have that uncanny knack for forgetting all about tact, introverts tend to think very carefully about everything. This means that the pros and cons of every decision are weighed, which means it is more likely they will make informed decisions. This type of thinking is great for dealing with personal and business situations. In fact, there have been studies that have shown that introverts are better at things like making music and playing video games. This is most likely due to thinking over every move they intend to make.

When it comes to technology, introverts use it a lot wiser than others do. For example, someone who is an introvert would not be likely to log onto their social media account and tell the entire world about every indiscretion they have ever made. While there are some introverted people that would use their account as a speaker, most others will not. Another good thing is the fact that they will be more likely to share useful information with others. While others are sharing memes, an introvert will share business news and other things they feel would be universally relevant.

Writing is a skill that is much easier said than done. While it is easy to put a pen on paper and allow words to fill the sheet, it is not simple to write something that others will find engaging and thought-provoking. Creating written magic requires a certain amount of inner creativity and deep thinking, and as you have been reading so far, this is something that comes quite naturally to an introvert. It is easier for people to do research and write a paper than it is to dig deep within yourself to create a masterpiece. Since introverts spend most of their time bonding with themselves, this is like second nature to them.

Being the victim of a crime is not something that can be prevented in many cases, but the way things are handled after are different for introverts and extroverts. While an extrovert will spend more time panicking about the situation at hand or trying to reason with their attacker, an introvert will take the time to observe the situation and mentally gather information that would be useful to law enforcement officers. So while and extrovert will describe their assailant as being overweight, tall and bearded, an introvert will have a better idea of his height, notice his limo and a tattoo on his wrist.

Have you ever tried to have a conversation with someone and it seemed like their minds were all over the place? Instead of having a thought-provoking chat, you may have felt like you had become witness to a verbal train wreck. This is not a common trait of introverts, so you would probably get more enjoyment out of having talked with them. While you may not glean as much information out of them as you would with someone else, there is a good chance that most of the information you are given will be deep and compelling. Again, this is tied to the thinking process that is quite unique to introverts.

When it comes to education, introverts are usually the ones that get the most out of their money. There are many people that enroll in colleges, then spend half of their time socializing and seeing how many parties they can attend before the semester is over. The reality is that introverts tend to have less friends, which is definitely not a bad thing. This means that they will most likely spend more time in the library than they will at frat parties. This tends to translate to better grades and more opportunities once they leave school and get out there into a more cutthroat world.

Romantic relationships tend to thrive when both partners believe that they are being listened to. In this sense, introversion can play a huge part in a successful union. If two introverts enter a relationship, chances are they will both know how to be attentive to the others' needs. The fact that most introverts listen more than they talk means that both parties will not battle one another for control of the microphone. They will be more likely to give the other one the stage sometimes and allow them to express themselves. As was stated earlier, introverts do not like to talk any more than they need to, so it will be easier for them to express themselves to their partners in as little words as possible. In fact, many introverts would rather write their feelings down and communicate that way.

Now that you have a clearer view into the mind of an introvert, it should be easy to see why this is a benefit more than a hindrance. If you have always been self-conscious about not being more out-there, you can relax now. As you can probably tell from reading all of the information above, there are lots of advantages to being an introvert, so you should embrace it.

Introverts and Dealing With Social Situations

For introverts, the best types of social situations are those where they can discuss ideas and concepts. They are generally not very good at social small talk and gossip, although they are much more comfortable if the gathering is a group of good friends that they have known for a long time. This is one of the few times introverts will open up and freely join the conversation because they are truly comfortable in this group of people.

When introverts are in a new social environment, they tend to keep to themselves or to a group of one or two people they know well. They may even have a conversation topic ready that they are comfortable discussing and you can be sure they have thoroughly thought through how it will play in this social situation. One of the great strengths of introverts is that they know how to ask great questions and how to really listen to the answers, so if there is a person to impress at a social function, an introvert is the one to do it.

Other introverts may be perfectly comfortable with one-on-one interaction during a social situation. They may enjoy large parties or social functions, but prefer sitting and watching all the people and the action from the sidelines. This may be a fun social event for an introvert. People watching instead of people interaction.

Being an introvert should not be confused with being a misanthrope. Most introverts actually enjoy others, however they typically favor quality over quantity in their friendships, choosing to create small, intimate circles of friends rather than large networks of acquaintances. In reality, it could be that introverts actually know their friends better because they have fewer to get to know.

Introverts who are shy might certainly have a difficult time in social situations. Even the introvert who is okay around people, but just doesn't want to do a lot of social mingling may be called upon to do it because of work or professional responsibilities.

For the shy introvert, these human interactions can be tough, because introverts would rather listen than talk and ask questions than answer. This makes it difficult to get to know another person.

For the shy introverts, there are some strategies that can help in these situations. Even the introvert who may deal with social anxiety in certain situations can use some of these tips to ease their fears.

• Just do it. Just get out there and network. Join organizations, talk to others in their business industry, and attend Chamber of Commerce events. The familiarity of the subject matter at these events will help break the ice and make it easier to get the conversational ball rolling.

As introverts, it is easier to discuss concepts and ideas, and since this is business, they are comfortable with the subject matter and from that subject, the conversation will naturally turn to other subjects.

They should force themselves to step outside their comfort zone as far as they can. They can even try using Twitter, Facebook, and LinkedIn to make new connections and increase their familiarity and relationships.

Individuals should push the boundaries of their comfort zones and try and meet new people at every event. They should try and learn something new each time and take home a new contact with each event as well.

Scientific studies in psychology show that when individuals interpret uncomfortable or difficult situations as challenges or adventures, they are better able to cope with the stress and anxiety, so just do it.

- Use social media. Almost every event puts their

program information on social media, so individuals can use this to get familiar with the people who will be attending upcoming social and networking events. They can also visit the venue to get familiar with the layout, parking, entrances, etc.

This may sound a bit weird, but the introverted individual should try watching a funny movie or television show ahead of time, too. This will get them in a happy mood and will carry over as they attend the event. They will radiate this positive, happy energy and this will invite people to get to know them.

• Set goals. Shy introverts should set some simple goals such as attending one networking or business social event a week and meeting one new business contact at each event.

Accomplishing these goals will help build their confidence and having these conversations and attending these business events will certainly help overcome their social anxiety, at least in these types of situations.

- Ask extroverted friends and colleagues for help. Most introverted people have extroverted friends and colleagues and if asked, these people will be glad to help. The introverted person can attend social events that they may not otherwise feel comfortable at with these friends. Once there, these friends and colleagues can help introduce the introvert to other people and start conversations.

Once at the event, the introverted person should not be intimidated if their extroverted friend begins to charm the room. The introverted individual should stand tall, smile, and be confident, while asking good questions and listening to the answers. This will also charm, but perhaps just one person at a time. That one person, however may be much more important than an entire room and the introvert should just be sure to get their contact information!

- Nerves can be good. Being nervous just means you are alive. Socializing is just like any skill. It takes practice. The shy introvert will get better and better the more they practice. The more they stretch their boundaries, the more adept they will get at the witty banter and repartee.

• It is about them, not you. This is really good advice. People love to talk about themselves, so when a situation is uncomfortable for the shy introvert, they should try taking the focus off themselves by asking questions and then listening closely and deeply to the other person's answers.

This helps them get to know the people they are talking with and helps the introvert become more comfortable opening up a bit about themselves as well.

These tips can help the shy introvert be more comfortable in those social situations that inevitably happen. Each step forward will help build their confidence in their own abilities as it builds their social and professional network at the same time. It is a win-win situation for this charming, but sometimes misunderstood personality.

How an Introvert Personality Can Be a Powerful Catalyst for Success

Success in life does not just belong to those that make the most noise or create the biggest stir. While many introverted people believe being soft spoken is a major liability, it can be a strength that is viewed as a reasonable and quiet reflective individual. In fact, speaking in a quiet tone, asking the right questions, and listening intently can create strong negotiators and powerfully successful people.

Like any other strategy for moving through life, introversion is actually a talent for navigating. Many of the most transformative individuals throughout history have been extremely introverted and shy. The list of these individuals would include Rosa Parks,

Eleanor Roosevelt, Charles Darwin, Frederic Chopin, Gandhi, Mother Teresa and especially Abraham Lincoln. Instead of focusing their attention on bolstering their egos, or believing that their introverted personality would work against them, they used their shy and reflective nature as an effective energy to create positive change.

Often times, our culture celebrates its hyperactivity and over-scheduling, where too much has to be done with too little time. We see the alpha approach as having the greatest value in society. However, it is often the individuals that are quieter in nature that are the most empowered. This is because their inner introvert personality provides the best environment for seeing the larger picture that is often found in solitude, silence and the inner strength required to achieve the best goals.

The Serious Conversationalist

Most individuals that have an introverted personality feel that chitchat is over-stimulating. It requires constantly jumping from one subject to another. Instead, an introvert tends to enjoy serious conversation with a deep focus on one topic that can be mutually shared with others with like interests. Studies indicate that individuals that partake in minimal amounts of small talk are likely to be happier because the conversations they engage in tend to be substantive.

A Solitary Path

Society tends to believe that the greatest achievements in life happen by committee. However, statistics indicate otherwise. Some of the largest leaps in life have been taken in solitude, where inventors, composers, writers, researchers and others have generated huge moves or shifts in the way that things are done when working all alone. In fact, brainstorming ideas tend to create only small shifts of

change for the better. Motivated and talented individuals tend to find their most creativity and efficiency when taking their creative journey on a solitary path.

Better Read

Social interaction is often considered to be

communicating directly one-on-one with individuals. However, some of the most successful individuals have been those that are well read. This type of social connection is usually a deeper and more fruitful communication. Introverted individuals tend to read more, and become significantly more empathetic with highly advanced social skills because they better understand social norms and the actions of others.

A Better Listener

Some of the most powerful individuals in the world are those that are better listeners. The actions of becoming a powerful effective leader are often a result of listening to those that are subordinate or under their command. In fact, introverted individuals often have good leadership skills because they are more likely to consider others' suggestions. Powerful introverts tend to work on their speaking skills more than extroverts and certainly smile much more. Being a better listener makes it easier to see the strength of others. It provides an easy course for encouraging subordinates to take a leadership role through their own initiative.

Recharging Batteries

Successful introverted individuals often act much like an extrovert whenever it is necessary. It is often an uncomfortable action of positively getting the message across in a dynamic way. However, this short burst of extrovert energy usually requires a recharge that often happens in a place of solitude. This is because the action of being "all out there" can be extremely over-stimulating to an introverted individual. Only by restoring or recharging their inner batteries can they clear their mind. In addition, falling back into natural introverted mode will provide access to deeper insights and feelings.

Achieving Goals

Power in an individual is often recognized as the one with the loudest voice. However, there is a certain subtle inner power of an introverted individual that is usually stronger and more intense. Through gentle tones and quiet words, insightful suggestions, creative ideas and thoughtful actions can move mountains.

Usually, successful introverts choose not to stand to speak the loudest. Instead, they strive to build alliances with others behind the scenes. Instead of speaking loudly about any problem, they simply chip away at it by themselves, or with their associates through skill, strategy and a plan of attack. It is important to remember that quiet persistence is a soft power that can move heaven and earth.

Embrace the Difference

Usually, an introverted individual understands that they are different from extroverts, who generally require ongoing stimulation. The introvert recognizes that quiet downtime is far more beneficial than dancing in the limelight. They often have wide ranging, deep differences that affect almost every aspect of daily living. Research indicates that an introverted personality is created by brain chemistry, which provides the ability to concentrate deeply and focus on one thing for an extended period. In fact, an introvert tends to have a long attention span.

Introverts have the ability to work extremely well alone. They are good at problem solving, listening, and forming very deep friendships. When compared to extroverts, they tend to have better interpersonal social skills and can be extremely talkative the moment they feel they are in a comfortable setting. However, they often lack the verbal spontaneity or social energy of an extrovert and are often drowned out at parties, meetings and social events.

In all, it is beneficial to embrace the difference from extroverts. The difference they experience might be socializing at a different pace than others, and taking the necessary time for self-reflection, rest and "alone" time. It is important to recognize that this is not antisocial behavior, just a specialized type of socializing.

Conclusion

Now that you have learned more about an introvert and what makes them tick, what can we say about them? Well, we can say that introversion should never be mistaken for shyness—granted there are shy introverts. Shyness is a condition and introversion is just who a person is. Shyness can be worked on to overcome it; being an introvert cannot. We can also say with great certainty that introverts are just as important and valuable to society as extroverts. Without the introverts helping to make wise and informed decisions, who knows what sort of chaos could ensue if extrovert made all the decisions!

We have learned that you can work on overcoming being shy. Social media outlets like LinkedIn, Twitter and Facebook are excellent examples of places to go to broaden one's network. These internet sites are just a few ways to push open the boundaries and help allow the shy person to feel more comfortable in social settings. Another way to overcome the shyness is to set goals for themselves. Go out and speak to someone new, even if it is to ask for the time or for directions. All that matters is that you are pushing yourself to do something you normally don't do. It's an experience that can feel daunting, but with enough time and practice, a shy introvert may feel more at ease in larger social settings. You will no longer be hiding away by yourself watching from the edges.

The Myers-Briggs Type Indicator is a simplistic and yet fascinating tool that can help you to determine where you fall on the introvert/extrovert scale. With only 4 simple questions to answer, there are 16 types that you could be. I suggest that if you are curious to know what type you are, go to http://www.myersbriggs.org to take the test for yourself. You'd be surprised by the results. They may offer a deeper perspective to your personality than you weren't even aware of. But

please, don't be saddened if you are labeled as an introvert though. You aren't condemned to a life of solitude! Remember, introverts often make good partners in relationships—both platonic and romantic—because they listen and do not struggle to be heard. If partnered with another introvert, your relationship may very well be a successful and fulfilling one!

Introverts aren't the sullen detached people tend to

think. We aren't dull and unintelligent, nor are we arrogant and anti-social. We enjoy people just as much as the next person. We find ways to entertain ourselves, often times with self-reflection and by creative avenues. We are the painters, the writers, the ones who prefer the backstage rather than the limelight. We are strong people who are aware of our surroundings and we are content with making tough choices because we have weighed out all the possible outcomes. As an introvert, we seek out the quiet corners in a noisy world in which we live in.

And to be honest, we are okay with that.